AN ELDER'S TAKE ON AGEING

Helen M Bryan

DEDICATION

They said, "Don't give up. You're not done. You can do this." So, I went on. I want to thank my own family, my DAS family and my Unity family for perfect support when I needed and asked for help. When I doubted, they were there.

PREFACE

During a weekend seminar my spiritual leader, Dennis Adams, acknowledged that he was a little upset upon age coming into his life—things were not as they used to be—his energy was different. Talking together during a break I said, "Just put yourself in *agreement*." "What did you say?", Dennis asked. I answered and told him all about my Energy/Activity Chart. His interest was such that he suggested I write a book and others wholeheartedly agreed. I was 89 almost 90 and really reluctant. Weeks passed and then I thought why not. I started. Thought it was complete. It wasn't. Added some more. Thought it was complete. It wasn't. There was still more. It's done. I'm finished. I hope you find this helpful.

TABLE OF CONTENTS

FORWARD

There is a simple trick to ageing. The simple trick is *agreeing*.

That's it!

If you know how to do that, read no more.

You've got it --- THE AGE *AGREEMENT*.

This little book is all about *agreeing* with ageing.

I mean, are you *agreeing* with ageing?

Are you really?

It doesn't matter how old you are now. Or before now. At some point in time (over years past) you looked in the mirror and were surprised.

What happened?

      Just yesterday I had no wrinkles.

      Just yesterday I had a beautiful head of hair.

Just yesterday I could work all day with energy in reserve to dance all night   and work the next day too.

Just yesterday I still felt young.

Just yesterday…. Remember now?

Age!   That's what happened.

Age!   It's got your attention.   You notice all the many little things you used to be able to do.   And you don't like it at all.

Upsetting? Yes!   Fearful? Yes!   Angry? Yes!   Denial? Yes!

Determined to stay young? Yes!   And the years go by.

How are you doing with the old age concept? Did you succeed in stopping the clock? Did you finally lose your cool? Did you find your answer? If so, please share it because I'm in the same boat you are.

Except, along the way, I learned a few tricks to help me keep my balance and prevent my getting lost or depressed.

<u>ONE</u>

The Age *Agreement*:

I like the word *agreement*. Being in *agreement* is a huge learning experience.

Agreeing puts you in harmony and allows you to stop fighting your mind and your body and to stop complaining about age.

Only by *agreeing* can you find willing acceptance which in turn allows you a good measure of peace.

> *Agreeing* puts you and age on the same side.

> *Agreeing* and accepting allows you to adjust to what is.

> *Agreeing* sees getting old from a different perspective with new possibilities.

> *Agreeing* opens up another way to explore life.

> *Agreeing* can mean opportunity instead of dwelling on past regrets.

So?

Learn to relax!

Let go!   Let God!

Love the new you just as you are!

TWO

Tricks to *Agreeing* begins with Story Time:

Every decade brings a change and a new challenge. Energy is a big one. Let me tell you my story about energy.

I was born in September in the year 1928. (I'll let you do the math.) Married when I was 23. Had four children (3 girls and a boy) by the time I was 27. Divorced when I was 36.

We lived in a substantial home on two acres in Franklin Village, Michigan. Circumstances necessitated that I continue working during the birth of my children and so called marriage. After my divorce, my ex fell short of any type of support so working was crucial. Thankfully, I did have my parents support as backup in every needed way.

In my late 40's after my kids were grown and away from home in college or married, I moved to a smaller house closer to Detroit, MI. At this new location, I started a vigorous routine every morning before going to work. It was either walking 1-2 miles or riding my bicycle 17 miles or swimming 1 mile at a local YWCA or jump roping or indoor exercising. Also, dancing every other night at different locations all over western Detroit and its suburbs. (Senior Singles. Live Bands. Loved it! Dancing was fun.) Sometime in my 50's I moved from Redford , MI. (a Detroit suburb) to a mobile park in Wixom, MI.

The years passed. I now had grandchildren in both Eastern and Western Michigan. Still single but now at 67 years old, I moved from Wixom to Grand Rapids, MI. into a small apartment in an independent senior building. I continued exercising daily before going to my new work place. Did all my own chores and driving all over the USA; East Coast, South, and cross country to California several times. I feel this history is necessary so you can understand where I'm coming from when I state that I've always been relatively healthy and active.

Then, all of a sudden, came the moment of truth. A 911 phone call. What happened that morning in April of 2015 was major surgery (GI Bleed) causing a complete blood exchange - 100%.

Hospital!   Rehab!   Home care!

 It took a long time to recover. Still, step by step, I managed steady fast improvement. The doctors and nurses attributed this growth to my being an ardent, energetic person who simply loved all types of physical activity. Amazing!

I kept on improving until months later when all of a sudden one day I went too far, did too much, and had a major setback.   What's that like?

Each set back consists of nausea, excruciating cramps, and just plain exhaustion. A set-back lasts 10-12 hours and two or more days before returning to so called normal.

This time my improvement was much, much slower. I found things I was able to do before surgery were no longer viable.   Rats!   Bugger all!

The improving and set-backs kept happening. Why?

My kids and I thought I had possibly become diabetic due to the stress of the GI Bleed. So, I went through the whole diabetic routine of blood tests, etc., etc. I began a diabetic support system, changed my diet, bought diabetic cook books and started keeping track of what I was eating. Then I discovered eating smaller amounts every three hours was more helpful than bigger meals three times a day.

Still, the improving then set-back, the up-down, the yo-yo affect kept happening.   Now what?

I had to keep exercising. This last time couldn't be blamed on diet.   Could it?   I was careful.   I was watching my diet.

Hopeless!   Confused!   Depressed!   Where did all the energy go?   I didn't know what to do or who to call and hated it.

So?   "Stop already, Helen."   Relax!   Pray!

And then an insight!   Perhaps!   Maybe!

It's silly but okay, I'll try it.

THREE

This is it!   An Energy/Activity Chart (EAC):

Take a full sheet of lined paper. Leaving three lines blank for titles, begin listing on the left side every weekly activity you do that requires effort plus energy to do it. Take one line for each activity like grocery shopping, laundry, driving, video exercise, walking, cooking, shower, cleaning, etc., etc. Then expand your list. For instance, shopping could be grocery shopping, clothes shopping, errands, etc. Some not major but still taking some energy like entertainment. List activities with others like playing cards or lunches in or out. Also list alone activities like jigsaw puzzles or water color painting or crayon art. Even fun activities take energy. Like going to the library or a birthday party or taking care of grand kids or even seeing a movie. I did not list reading or watching TV or going to church because these activities are resting to me.

You make your own list as simple or detailed as you want.

Over this list title ACTIVITIES. Now on the right side of your paper draw two vertical lines for columns. Over both of these columns put the title ENERGY USED.   Under this title but over the first column write USUAL. Over the second column write MORE.

Next, by your own standards and to the right of each activity, assign a number representing the energy used by you to accomplish it. Remember that your list will be appropriate to your age and life style.

Following are two examples. The first is my simple original Energy/Activity Chart. Remember I'm almost 90 now. I did this first chart of mine when I was 88. I'm almost a genuine Elder and proud of it. (I think I have to be 90 to be genuine.)

Let's begin.

Make your chart. List various activities, make your columns and assign a usual value to the energy this activity takes for you to accomplish it.

I have taken the liberty here to show you my original Energy/Activity Chart known as EAC throughout this booklet.

ORIGINAL ENERGY/ACTIVITY CHART		
ACTIVITIES	**ENERGY USED**	
	Usual	More
Shower / washing my hair	1.5	
Laundry bi-weekly & changing bed sheets	3	
Grocery shopping bi-weekly	2	3
Driving my car 20 miles	1	
Card playing w/ friends (average 1.5 hours)	1	2
Eating out w/friends or family (average 1.5 hours)	1	2
Walking 20 minutes	2	
Video-exercise	1	2

Looking at my example above you can see that I listed only those I was already aware of that took some energy to do. To me energy used produced tiredness. Hence, I based my chart values on tiredness and with that in mind applied points from one to four (1–4).

Following is a pie graph of the same example as this page. Hopefully seeing the EAC as a pie graph will allow a better understanding of my following point explanation.

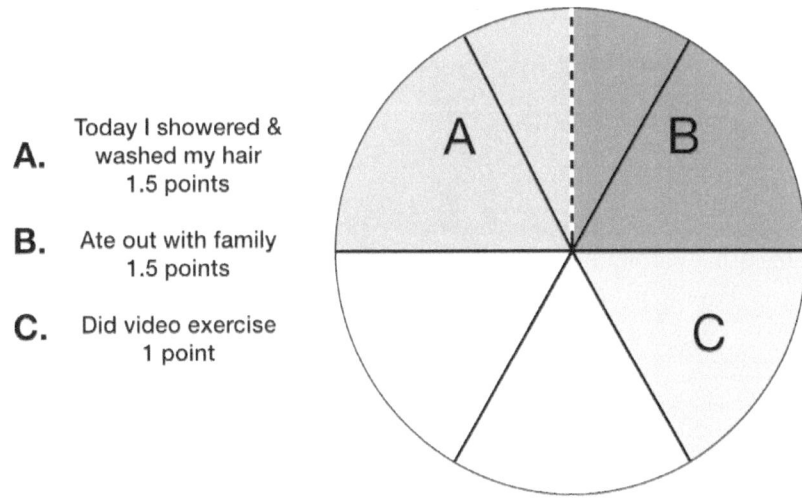

A. Today I showered & washed my hair
1.5 points

B. Ate out with family
1.5 points

C. Did video exercise
1 point

Continuing: In the beginning I found if I limited myself to 4 points of consumed energy then 4 points became a perfect day. If I went up to 5 points, I was still okay. At 6 points (almost too much), I needed to watch it. If I went as high as 7 points, I was in trouble and paid for it.   How?   I became way too tired. The dreaded yo-yo! The next day or two or three precipitated cramps, major pain, and nausea. My beginning three point range was 4-5-6. But life kept improving. Soon my three point range became 5-6-7 and then went up to 6-7-8. Doing too much (going over my range) still meant deep trouble. And yes, you guessed it. The yo-yo once again. Knowing all this helped me to gradually expand my EAC point system and improved my overall health vitality and emotions.

FOUR

Explanation of my value/point system:

As seniors I assume each of us has been to the Doctor or hospital. If you're having any pain they ask you "on a scale of 1–10 what is your pain level, 10 being the highest and 1 being the lowest. Give me a figure. If it's no pain, what is it? Is it stress? Is it tiredness? From 1-10 what is it?"

Try this method to arrive at your own point values. And by the way what criteria are you basing your point values on? Is it stress or pain or tiredness or something else?

Each one of you must determine for yourself how tired you get doing something and then give it a value. Use that one activity as your base and compare the others to it.

I chose grocery shopping and then I recognized it was a sliding scale based on time taken, quantity needed, did I have to ask for help because I couldn't find what I wanted and even was there a long line at check-out.

After making your list, go over it and add-up-only-those-points-from-the-activities-you-did-that-day.

What have you discovered?   Where are you?
When do you need to stop and regroup?

Maybe you need to take a nap.

What's your range?

EXTENDED ENERGY/ACTIVITY CHART POINT SYSTEM

ACTIVITIES	ENERGY USED
Shower and washing hair	1.5
Doing laundry/changing bed sheets	3
Shopping: grocery (average 1.5 hours)	2-3
" clothes	1-3
" mini grocery or dollar store	1
Driving my car 20 miles	1
Playing card games (1 hr.=1 pt.) (2 hrs.=2 pts.)	2
Eating out with friends (average 1.5 hrs.)	1-2
Walking outdoors 1 mile or 20 minutes	2
In house exercise 25 min. entire program	2
Attending church w/social coffee after service	1

Facilitating "A Course in Miracles" class at church	1
Adult crayon-art pictures – usual 2 hrs.	2
Water color painting—usual 1 hr.	3
Playing piano – usual 1 hr.	1
Crochet – usual 1 hr.	1.5
Diabetes Class, 1 hr.	1
Jig-saw puzzles – usual 3 hrs.	2
Library	1
Grandchildren's birthday parties	4
Baby Sitting	4

Add-only-those-points-from-activities-used. Again to me, 4 points is a perfect day, 5 is OK, 6 is too much, 7 means I'm in deep trouble.

Is all this helpful? Do you have questions? Let's answer a few.

Question: What if I want to do something extra like washing my windows?

Answer: I stop doing other things so I have the energy needed to accomplish this special task. Likewise, if I want to do something extra in the evening, I save energy points in the morning by staying quiet and peaceful.

Question: I don't live by myself. I room with my children so I don't do groceries, cleaning, laundry or cooking. What should I list?

Answer: List what affects you. Does noise affect you? Does stress affect you? How about going to the dentist or doctor? What about entertainment activities like going to a grandchild's school event? Obviously your list would be different than mine. You get to list your own activities and apply the value points to them.

Question: Is this EAC somewhat similar to the way one keeps track of calories or sugar or carbohydrates, fat, protein or salt?

Answer: Yes. It is similar but it's still a matter of disciplining yourself until it's familiar.

Question: Is it complicated?

Answer: No. It's simple because it's a feeling level and it's yours. You choose.

When I first explained my EAC to my daughters they heard me but didn't pay too much attention. But my son was impressed and very supportive and encouraging. Now they all can tell by my phone voice how I am feeling and where I'm at. They ask what point I've been on lately. A side note here: I've noticed that my daughters tend to protect me from overdoing while my son encourages me to keep on doing. "Don't give up just try again."

 An EAC of your own may work. Just try it.   You may find that you like it.

FIVE

Another story learning about *agreeing*:

This brings me to what happened a decade back while I was on vacation with my family. My daughter's family has a cottage on Russell Island off the South Channel between Algonac, Michigan and Canada in the St. Clair River. There are no cars on the island and it necessitates a very short ferry ride from Algonac to the island. Then we walk, bicycle or golf cart to the cottage. The river connects Lake St. Clair and Lake Huron. Big lake freighters, ocean freighters and ocean liners pass right by. The water is usually 69 degrees and is very cold, very deep (70' in the middle of the channel) and has a swift current. There is a local swimming dock from shore to deep water. The point of my story is as follows:

My girls were concerned about my swimming alone because of my age (late 70's) and asked me to promise them I wouldn't go swimming without someone with me. I did promise. Yes, I did. BUT the next day was very hot. I was very hot. I wanted to take a dip. They were not around. Oh yes, I remembered that I had promised. So I walked out on the dock in my shorts and tank top, took off my flip-flops and climbed down the slanted ladder until my lower legs where in the nice cold water. While still hanging on the ladder with my right hand I proceeded to have some fun while I was cooling off.   I was there quite a while just swinging my feet. Enjoying myself.   Playing. Then something compelled me to look up to the dock. I saw two feet firmly planted there. I looked further up and guess what? There stood my daughter with hands on her hips, "Mo-o-ther! You promised." (You know the sound.)

"I'm not swimming," I said.

"You promised!" was the response.

Heatedly I replied, "I'm not swimming!"

She protested and said, "You could slip on those slippery steps, lose your balance, fall, hit your head and no one's around. You could die of hypothermia."

Very emphatically I came back with, "I did promise. I'm not swimming. I'm perfectly capable of watching out for myself. I'm not a child. Go away."

She did and eventually I calmed down, climbed out and went back to the cottage.

A few days later while driving home together (daughter's driving), I said that I had a thought during the night; "Children from birth on are encouraged to stretch themselves just a little more. Each advance is praised and further advance is lovingly encouraged. So children advance best under the influence of praise and love, always one step up and then another. Just the opposite happens with us seniors. We start moving down identical to the way children move up and it's most always under some type of fear, hopelessness, abandonment, etc. You name it. We see pity and hurt-for-us in the eyes of relatives and friends as they watch little things slide away— things that we can no longer do.   Is there a way to appreciate and praise parents letting go the same way we did our kids as they were stepping up?

"Why can't you encourage me in every step that I take which I recognize and adjust to?   Say, "Well done, Ma, or good for you."   That would be helpful because it's hard letting go.   It's a whole new learning process."

She heard me (God bless her) but also said it was up to me to recognize and give credit to myself. I heard her too and I had to acknowledge that. We both took time to absorb this and then we let it pass.

Food for more thoughts regarding seniors moving down (declining) identical to the way kids move up (advancing); What is also obvious is that the kids are always a step ahead of the parent. (Parents are always in a catching-up-to-them phase.) Likewise, seniors are a step ahead in their decline and their children have not expected or anticipated the down-trend. OR, do the children of seniors wish to be relieved of the burden of their ageing parents – no time – too busy with their own kids – and their own lives. ??

Elders are all about learning how to let go. Some do it graciously and some fight to the end. The cry is "Give me a reason to live!"

In case you missed it, this is also a trick. *Agreeing* is being aware of today's circumstances which is really nothing but understanding the ageing process.

SIX

EAC One Month Before 90:

September 1, 2018, fifteen days before I'm 90, three and a half years since my 911 call and approximately two years since I started my original Energy/Activity Chart. This means that my EAC needs to be up-dated.

I'm on vacation at Russell Island again. I love the water. That's why I had to come. It's so clear. It's so cold. It's also so deep. It draws me. I wish I could still dive right in. That's so tempting but irresponsible. Today I walk down the slanted ladder very slowly. Only letting my feet get used to it before I go one step more and again one step at a time ever so carefully until I can let go of the ladder and immerse myself in the cold refreshing water. Not over my head yet, still too soon. Oh my! That feels so good. And I'm swimming! Well, to be honest, only treading water and only for five or six minutes. It's cold! Tomorrow I'll stay in longer and attempt swimming against the current. Can I? Tomorrow?

Guess what? This is the third day of my vacation and I was able to swim against the current about 20 feet and even dove head first off the dock. Eureka!   I also stayed in the water at least 15 minutes—maybe a bit longer than that. Wow! Of course, as I promised, I was not alone. Two of my daughters were with me.

Did you wonder how I would write my EAC today?

First of all the essentials just so I know how much energy I have to begin with. It's different at the cottage. Consider that on my original EAC there was no need for me to list minimal walking or points for stairs because my apartment is a little less than 400 sq. ft. For instance here there are four steps that get me from the ground to the porch. So that's 1 point because I go up and down all the day long. And there are distances between the bathroom and the kitchen and several steps between the various rooms again which I don't have In my apartment. So that's 1 point. And there's 50 feet average from the cottage to the water, maybe 70 feet further to go out on the dock. And I have to consider all the many times I've been leaving the cottage to go outside. I must give that 2 points. Don't forget sitting and eating outside all day long. This is different also and deserves another 1 point. Stay with me now as I look at my EAC here at Russell Island vacation day six:

Essentials as stated above amount to:	5 points
Swimming and playing in the water 20 minutes with slanted ladder down to the water and back up:	4 points
I swept the porch this morning while waiting for my daughter as she was walking around the island. No porch at my place and I can't remember the last time I used a broom. Shouldn't have done it, too tiring so it deserves	5 points
And then we spent some time on a jigsaw puzzle	2 points
Also helped make new Potato Chip Cookies and a Lemon Tart	1 point
Essentials totaled makes	17 points

Did I overdo? You bet. Did I pay for it? You bet. It set me back two full days. Instead of 12 hours of cramps this time it took from 7 PM overnight until noon of the next day and, of course, complete rest, minimal eating and I only got to taste the crumbs of the Lemon Tart. The rest was all gone. I ask you, was that fair?

Yes, I wasn't paying attention to my Energy/Activity Chart at all. Yes, I wasn't listening to myself and all because I was having fun and feeling good and wanting to be part of good times with my family.

All this writing about the necessity of doing my part (trying to keep up) was because if I'm no longer useful how can they love me? I felt tears come to my eyes. I knew I'd gotten triggered into an old fear. What fear? Feeling unworthy that's what. (As I knew it, love was conditional.)

Oh my! I had to turn this around. Because you can't go back. I know that. If you do, you must face it—learn from it—and then let it go. Acceptance is the key. I know that. You won't accept what you fear. I know that too. So I chose to face this underlying fear of mine. I felt I should not and must not ask my girls "Why do you love me?" They'd be shocked. They'd want to know where-did-that-come-from?

Help! What do I do now? And then I thought of my Mom.

How did I love my Mom? My answer was without any conditions. That's how. It was so simple. I just loved her. And when she got old I enjoyed helping her in any way I could to make her life a little happier and easier.

Here I am myself older, still trying to keep up. I guess it's my turn to enjoy my girls loving, protecting and helping me. They really want to. And somehow, I must simply learn how to embrace all this caring.

Have I listened to all that I've been writing here? No. BUT I'll keep trying and soon I will. It's really never outside yourself. What goes around, comes around. Change of attitude here I come.

Agreeing with ageing is hard. Someone once said, "Growing old isn't for sissies." Life is still an endless learning process. When you think you know it all and you've finally got it, watch out. Right around the corner you find out you didn't know it at all.

This is a quote I found in (CIM) Miracles magazine. "You only live once, but if you do it right, once is enough." --Mae West

SEVEN

Looking further:

Agreeing can become a way of life. Especially these days as technology keeps upgrading on us. For seniors it's happening so fast it's very hard to keep up.

Every time I turn around someone's upgraded my cell phone. That means another way to go. When I was a kid once you learned something it stuck and stayed with you for years and years. Not so today. The work place has changed. Peer groups are the rage with new rules. Competition seems fiercer than ever. Grocery store layouts change every time you turn around. Clothes are arranged by color instead of size with every size in that design on the same rack.

Or, no more shopping in stores because the current trend is buying using the internet. Choose several styles and have them sent to you. Try them on in your own home. If you don't like them, send them back without charge. Woe unto you if you don't have a computer. Now you can buy theater tickets for the movie you want, the day, the seat and the time you want and go directly in. No lines. WOW!

And what about open marriage or don't get married at all. Just live together. That's a whole new ball game.

I'm upset. I don't understand. I get mightily confused. My attitude must change. Being defensive does not work. It closes me down. What we resist, persists.

Agreeing instead of resisting or becoming angry is the only way to go. Otherwise, the old rocking chair is just around the corner and very enticing.

How about you?

Are you with me?

EIGHT

Resistance to Ageing:

Let's talk a little about our resistance to the whole ageing process.

A big hindrance to *agreeing* with ageing is usually attachment. Attachment is simply refusal to let go. I implore you to deeply search yourself.

Can this be true?

Are you attached to responsibility or commitment, personal identity or love or allegiance? You name it.   Or could it be something as simple as you still want the good-old-days.   Are we as seniors or elders stagnated in the way it was in the good-old-days?

The First Commandment is "Thou shalt have no other Gods before Me." What does that mean? One of our biggest attachments (another God) is family; spouse, children, parents, a significant other, a job, a calling, friends, life itself. You name it.

Life itself is so precious to us that we are programmed to save life at any cost. Looking below that feeling of saving life at any cost (that program) is fear and because we don't know what's beyond, we won't (not can't) but won't let go. And perhaps we won't even trust or believe in God enough to let go.

This clinging to attachments is also clinging to the past. There is comfort in the past. We know our past. What's ahead of us, the unknown, is fearful. Very fearful, and we refuse to let ourselves move into it gracefully. Instead of peace, *agreeing to the ageing process*, we fight ageing endlessly.

This is how I look on fear.

Fear is a false God. And this false God is mighty. To protect this fear-God from over-whelming me, I erect walls around it to stop it from escaping. (When will I not see that all my energy goes to keeping fear contained?) My walls that keep fear in also keep me away from love and forgiveness.

So what will I chose? Will I erect walls to contain this fear-God or will I open myself, let fear escape, and embrace the love which I feel now and always have felt, unknowingly perhaps, but ultimately still true.

As written in "A Course In Miracles" from the Foundation of Inner Peace: "You make what you defend against, and by your own defense against it, is it real and inescapable. Lay down your arms, and only then do you perceive it false."

Who am I really? A jailor or a free spirit? A jailor chained by the very fear I'm trying to escape from or a free spirit releasing my fear chains and embracing the love, wonder and joy of freedom.

Like I've said over and over again: Peace can only come with *agreement.*

AGREEING WITH THE AGE I'M IN.

If you think about it, ceasing to *agree* with where we really are keeps us from living today.

Letting go allows us to live life. Fighting hard to live is just the opposite. Fear tightens every cell In our body so that living-life (oxygen) can't get through and our immune system goes way down making us susceptible to colds, illness and depression.

What are you still clinging to? Is the ultimate fear our own immortality? Can we, will we, put ourselves in the hands of God?

Agreeing with that premise, can we now enjoy this day?   Be fully and completely in the light of this moment?

NINE

Another little trick to ageing:

I said earlier that I needed to change my attitude. It's really simple if you choose to do it. Think of yourself by another name. For instance, "I'm not old. I'm an elder."

According to the American Century Dictionary:

> Old means (1) advanced in age not young or new, (2) made long ago, (3) long in use, (4) worn, dilapidated or shabby from age or use
>
> Elder means (1) senior—of greater age, (2) persons older and usually venerable
>
> Venerable means entitled to respect on account of character, age, etc.

According to Roget's International Thesaurus:

> Old refers to ancient, past, former, senile
>
> Elder refers to older, senior, veteran, church
>
> Venerable refers to old, estimable, sage

Which would you prefer? Being old and dilapidated or being an Elder entitled to respect, a sage, estimable. In some societies the Elder is revered.

I'm an Elder and proud of it.

TEN

Agreeing makes a Lighter YOU:

Don't forget that Ageing Demands Patience. Whew! That's a big word. Patience!

An elder friend of mine said this to me because I was being impatient. She said that her husband was just like me and she had to remind him over and over that, "Patience is a virtue." And that "Diversity brings patience." (Bible quotes.)

Patience has never been in my vocabulary. Why? Because I'm a Virgo. Virgo's demand organization and discipline and perfection. Yes, we're very loving but extremely hard (critical) on ourselves.

Accepting help is so humbling. How does one do it? With patience. With love. With honor both to others and to ourselves. It's our turn to make someone else's day by letting them help us.

Do you remember holding the door for someone who took longer than you to get through? Was he or she older or on a walker or crutches? You held that door for them with patience and a genuine smile. Now that smile and patience needs to be given to ourselves as we take longer than before to accomplish a task, even a simple task.

We are still doing a good turn. It's just from the other side. Look at life this way. Everyone is right. From their experience they are right. Agreed?

I agree being a senior or an elder is not for sissies. Surprisingly it's become the happiest part of my life. Now I'm all about unconditional love. No judgment on me or others as much as I can. Just allow. Listen. Don't give advice unless asked and only answer specifically what is asked. Stop. Do not go on and on. Say no more unless asked again.

Remember in all of this *agreeing with ageing* we must still respect the boundaries of those who are still in need of boundaries and not offer more than can be received.

So, Follow the KISS principal. "Keep it short and simple."

Am I still learning? You bet!

I try not to take things personal because it really is not outside myself.

Every relationship is a learning experience. Even

my relationship with inanimate things like my four-wheel-walker and my car. My walker's name is Charlie because he's independent and only helps me when I need it. My car's name is My Lady because she's mature and always on the lookout, has eyes in the back of her head and keeps me safe. Why do I name them? Just because it makes me smile.

It's been said that your car is your therapist. I believe that. Several times over the years my car has stopped me from accidents—moved me out of the way. So, yes, I believe in my car. I believe God is in all things. Many times I've gotten lost in thinking as miles and time have gone by without my being present. My car did it's own driving. Just imagine that! Admit it. It's not just me. I know you've experienced this. I talk to my car all the time and she listens to me without judging. Sometimes I ask My Lady if she talks to her comrades (motor buddies) and if she does, what do they talk about? Enough said about that.

From my viewpoint, what else can I say that would be helpful to you? On the other hand, we are all different in personalities and experiences. Would you be my friend and listen to me some more?

ELEVEN

Facing myself:

Today five months later, I need to make myself a revised Energy/Activity Chart because after hitting that 17 point day when I was on my two week Island vacation I wound up in the hospital with Colonic Stricture Surgery. They cut out and repaired previous scar tissue which was restricting feces flow, removed the right side of the colon and reattached the small intestine to healthy tissue. I'm still recovering and trying to recognize this new me. Look below.

Activities	Points
Cards limited to 1.5 hrs. or less & a few times a week only	2-3
No night time activity	0
No commitments they drain energy	0
Laundry takes 3 hours including changing bed sheets	5
Grocery days increase because it's time limited	2-3

Drug store is added as an alternate	1
I can't help others like before. I must come first now.	2-3

> Example: Airplane oxygen/mask usage. I'm accepting help now. I'm the one in need. I don't like it and it takes energy because I'm resistant & reluctant.

Depression takes lots of energy	5-8
Getting up facing the day	1-4
Friends and lunches out	2
Jig-Saw Puzzles	3-4
Shower & washing my hair	2

As you can see from what I've listed under activities, I'm in no condition to make a chart. I think I'm still in recovery from the operation. I can't concentrate as before and therefore have no idea how to even begin establishing a range of points. Rewriting this only keeps me in the doldrums.

I need to renew myself. I need to see myself in a new positive way. Perhaps I'll re-read what I've written about *agreeing*.

What do I desire?   Rainbows.   Sunshine. Flowers.   Hope.

I need to know I'm still worthy and needed.

I want God's peace!

This is not relevant to my EAC but, here is a fun fact:

Did you know that one minute of anger weakens the immune system for four or five hours? On the other hand, one minute of laughter boosts the immune system twenty four hours. Something to think about.

TWELVE

Re-Reading What I Wrote:

There are several revealing hidden secrets in what came up as I began writing this book. That's one thing beneficial in keeping a journal. You have the ability to uncover a deep fear you had stuffed way down inside of you. One you didn't want to acknowledge. One that meant too much—hurt too much—frightened you too much to admit to. For me it came up in Chapter Five. A cry, "Give me a reason to live."   I must own that cry.

When I was younger my ex and I had stopped in a tavern for lunch and a beer. On the wall behind the bar was this sign. "FREE BEER TOMORROW" Never forgot that. It made me laugh then and makes me laugh now to remember it.

We all know that tomorrow never comes. And, of course, one reason to live is we're not dead yet. Without an answer to my cry and in that then-moment-of- time, I just became quiet.

We don't really know what we can do.

While I was on a spiritual weekend retreat with Dennis Adams, he along with some of my friends there, encouraged me to write a book about ageing. Going back home I thought about it but it scared me. Who me?

It took about two weeks and then in my dreams I think (NO, I know) I was inner-directed by God to uncover this particular deep- seated fear. I woke up with the clear thought, "Helen, write a book about ageing!" And so I did and still am writing this book.

I've always loved to write. I kept and still do keep a journal. I guess it's kind of a hobby. Why don't you try it? Put yourself *in agreement* to be willing to up-lift yourself. Put yourself in *agreement* to be willing to develop a hobby. Let's name some possibilities here.

Volunteer in something that interests you. Get involved in politics. Do something you didn't have time to do before like water-color or oil-painting. Keep it simple. Try pencil or crayon-art instead. Become a finish-carpenter. Construct a ship in a bottle. Build kites. Putter with clay and mold something beautiful.

Whatever held you back before NOW is your time to LET-IT-GO. If you're physically handicapped, can you use that handicap to inspire yourself and others?

I guess it's about learning to love ourselves unconditionally. Remember that *AGREEING* IS THE BRIDGE BETWEEN DENIAL AND ACCEPTANCE.

Study the stars. Become spiritual. Strum a guitar. Try fishing. Perfect your golf. Consult with your cousins and build a family tree. If you've always dreamed of traveling and now don't have the money, go to your local library and dream travel by reading all about the world we live in. Become a history buff. Create a herb garden.

Stop feeling sorry for yourself. When you've hit rock bottom pick yourself up. See yourself happy. Happiness is a habit. Take some time to cultivate it. Remember the joy times and go from there. If you don't remember any joy times, pretend as if you do and go from there. Let your imagination take over. All you need is faith in as little as a mustard seed.

Only the present time is where your life is. If you would be a joy and a light to others you must first be a joy and a light to yourself.

Life is a mystery. Find yourself. Know who you are. Look in the mirror, say your name out loud and tell yourself, "There you are. Hi! Welcome home!" Smile.

We each have the ability to be truthful and to know and accept ourselves and own both what we like and what we don't like. We each have the ability in faith and love to say NO if it's not in our best interest or if we simply don't want to. We each have the ability to reveal ourselves to others and thus receive like truthfulness and love to come back.

In therapy we say, "I can only know that much of myself that I have the courage to share with you."

Keep calm and be crazy, laugh, love and live it up because this is the oldest you've been and the youngest, you'll ever be again.

THIRTEEN

Worthiness:

Agreeing with ageing keeps me open. Wherever there is openness there is hope.

In Chapter Six I used the word unworthy. It surprised me because during my lifetime I never questioned if I was needed. Others around me were in the same boat I was. We were measured by our accomplishments-–what we did. One of the fallacies of age is that we no longer belong. We are no longer needed. Our families have grown away from us on-their-own and we've been retired either willingly or unwillingly. It's a quandary that's put us on this quest to find ourselves. Who we are and who we are not.   Are we worthy?

Remember that God doesn't make junk.

It's a fallacy to even contemplate we could be little in any way. We must guard our thoughts judiciously because whatever we think becomes real-–what we believe becomes true for us. Therefore, cultivating a hobby is well worth doing because it can bolster (prop-up, encourage) that need to be needed—to still feel worthy.

This basic value of ourselves seems to come up all the time. Every time we don't get what we want there it is again. Does it remind you of childhood? The terrible twos? It's when we were first told NO. Within your mind is the question, "Why don't they love me anymore?"

In the children's book, Skin Horse Tells Rabbit: "that by the time one becomes REAL most of your hair has been loved off, and your eyes drop out and you get all loose in the joints and very shabby. But these things don't matter at all because once you are REAL you can't be ugly, except to people who don't understand."

The truth about ourselves is we are worthy simply because we are. I don't have to prove myself. I am worthy just as I am.

Let go of what others have said or how you think they see you now. You are in charge of your life. YES! You are! Believe it! Think it! Know it!

Don't let yourself get in your own way. Go out. Get a haircut. Get a massage. Dress the part of success. You really know all this. Why have you let yourself forget? What do you get out of giving

up? Do you like sympathy? "Oh, you poor kid."
You do know it takes more muscle to frown than it
does to laugh don't you?

Besides laughter begets laughter.

Mingle with those who make you laugh. Smile a
lot. Remember some of the good times when you
played a prank and got away with it or saw a
double rainbow or watched over a new-born. Did
you ever watch a mother cat give birth to her
kittens? Find something that gives you joy and
says to you, "I'm still worthy. I don't have to
please anyone else but me. I can be outrageous in
my old age and wear mismatched socks with
impunity."

DEPEND ON NO ONE BUT YOURSELF FOR THE
LOVE YOU NEED!

What do you believe in? Is it God? Then live the
life of love. Don't let anyone make you feel you're
not enough just as you are.

As I write all this, I realize I'm also talking to
myself. You can plainly see the ups and downs I
go through. It's also very clear to me re-reading
this book, that I'm exactly where I'm supposed to
be at my age. What I'm going through is typical.

Questioning myself—rethinking myself—
bolstering myself—looking for answers.

You might say I recycled myself—or recreated me.
I resisted as long as I could but eventually the
electronic age captured me too. I'm exercising my
mind and my psyche. "Eureka, Helen! Well
done!"

I feel excited and daring and young again.

I've listened to my heart, forged ahead and met
the challenge.

FOURTEEN

The Healing Process:

There's so much to be said about healing. Putting myself in *agreement* with the healing process involves both negative and positive thoughts and come to think about it both sides are equally powerful. So, let's begin this chapter by taking the fear away and looking at healing objectively.

Recently I came across a documentary on Netflix titled "HEAL" whose primary approach was holistic methods for healing. The following is what I heard and took notes on. The documentary states that the medical approach deals primarily with trauma, infection, emergency, and acute illness. It does not deal with the unknown symptoms. The holistic approach for healing deals with mind, body, emotion and energy. The documentary shows personal histories of people from all walks of life and varied ages with difficult physical, mental and emotional health problems. The network also incorporated people from all aspects of the many healing professions with their opinions, facts and experiences on the human psyche and physical health. Some of their findings show that there are six elements that forecast sickness:

These are: (1) Accumulation which produces heat In the body and may show up simply as excessive belching; (2) Aggravation which now shows up as heartburn; (3) it Spreads, the accumulation looking to find a home; (4) Localization, actually finding and going to the weakest part of the body; (5) Disease, for example arthritis; and finally, (6) Diversified, meaning further expansion or, using the same example, now becoming rheumatoid arthritis. The way to stop the progression of the disease is to start ridding yourself of the Accumulation.

Still speaking from the documentary "HEAL" we note the following. "There are nine attributes to healing. They are: (1) Radically changing your diet; (2)Taking control of your health; (3) Following intuition; (4) Using herbs and supplements; (5) Releasing suppressed emotions; (6) Increasing positive emotions; (7) Embracing social support; (8) Deepening spiritual connection; and (9) Having a strong reason for Living. What's involved in healing isn't just food. You'll note that only two of the nine resort to physical healing. The other seven resort to mental, spiritual and emotional healing. Belief itself heals.

Accept. Believe. Surrender. Relax.

LET GO of whatever it takes to accomplish emotional freedom. Fight and flight or rest and repair. Choose. If you believe it, you can achieve it.

On the positive side of healing are six elements beginning with: (1) Forgiveness which generates healing; (2) Meditation to relieve stress; (3) Imagination to visualize complete health; (4) a deep dedication to Faith and Trust; (5) Gratitude to give thanks; and (6) an ability to Focus on life and to remember the Mission is complete remission.

So, thoughts and beliefs affect our health. Held emotions, of which 90% are caused from stress, create destiny in our bodies. Our bodies are intelligent. Everything starts in the mind. Toxic thoughts produce toxic symbols. We need to remember that the power of love which made the body can also heal the body. We are the architect of our own being. We need to change our mind from fear to love and then, all we have to do is get-out-of-the-way.

Healing is obsessive to the degree that our obsessiveness keeps the fear and pain of sickness very much alive. Following your heart, common sense, is simply forgetting about it. Put it all in the hands of God, rest, relax, and enjoy your day.

Ask yourself, "What am I getting out of being sick? If you've been hanging on to sickness because it keeps your family coming around (this is just one reason) then you need to forgive yourself for this manipulative control. You might ask, "How do I do this?"

The book, A Course in Miracles, says that "Forgiveness is an empty gesture unless it entails correction. Without this, it is essentially judgmental rather than healing."

I firmly believe that *AGREEING* HELPS FAST PHYSICAL HEALING.

So what do you say? What's your state of mind? Do you want to improve your health? Do you want to get well? Do you believe in healing? Are you ready to be healed? How willing are you to be healed? If your answer to each of these questions is YES, then speak and act in line with healing. Know you have already received it and YOU HAVE. GIVE THANKS! LET GO!

There's a song that always pops up in my mind. It's, "Our thoughts are prayers and we are always praying. Our thoughts are prayers. Be careful what you're saying."

I am well aware that it is easier to give love than to ask for it. I am well aware that it takes much energy, intent and dedication to change. I am well aware that it takes wholehearted effort.

Don't be afraid. Don't give up. Have FAITH. GOD always works to our highest good. Sometimes that's different than what we think we need or want.

Still, just believe and it is already accomplished.

FIFTEEN

Positive Affirmations that help the principals of *Agreeing with Ageing*:

There are many needed affirmations throughout this book but I still would like to present you with a few more. Find those that speak to you?

Today I LET GO and LET GOD.

    I am well, whole and complete.

I view my world with appreciation and wonder.

    I look forward to new changes in my life.

Sharing brings more caring and information.

    I am willing to follow my heart.

I own a positive attitude. Today I will laugh a lot.

    Today I choose to see this situation in a new way.

Appearances are temporary impressions and not an accurate picture of me.

    My highest thought is always available.

Today I WILL to exercise my mind body, my emotional body and my soul body.

> I free myself today from any thought of lack or limitation.

I am grateful that the future I desire is in the process of manifesting now. "Thank You, God."

> I'm not the only one. I am not alone.

I have the power of Spirit within and the ability to make a lasting difference in my world.

> I am the light that I need and I let it shine, let it shine, let it shine.

I am confident and secure that I can and will be successful.

> I welcome a spirit of play—a childlike wonder, curiosity and delight in all that I do.

Agreeing means achieving. I want peace.

Charles Fillmore, a co-founder of Unity, wrote "I am alive, alert, awake, joyous and enthusiastic about my life." This is a solid wakeup affirmation but if it's too much try "Fake it 'till you make it."

Bill Diedrich, a Unity speaker, facilitator of "A Course In Miracles" as well as "A Course Of Love", and writer of several self-help books says, "I am mindful of my emotional state. I direct my thoughts and emotions toward Love, healthy growth, and healing. I move through the darkness of fear and into the Light of Love."

SIXTEEN

Left Alone:

This is a huge issue for elders and it's one each of us has had to handle time after time during our lives. Is it facing you now?

My friends, even family, are leaving either making their transition or giving up being independent and moving in with their children or into a final ageing facility. This type of adjustment happens more frequently now. I myself am the only living parent on both sides of my four children and their spouses which makes me also the only living grandparent. My kids and grandkids are extending themselves outward in all kinds of ways---in distance, in knowledge, and in experience.

There's nothing I can do about any of this except just keep myself out-of-the-way, make no judgment either for or against, stay happy for them and bless them all to their greatest good.

That part's the first step. But when I'm alone and my brave front has disappeared, old fears and resentments about abandonment and rejection pop up. These events are personal to me and when I was younger I had my ways of coping. But now it all feels too immense. I don't want to fall apart or become hugely depressed so . . . .

How do I clear it out of my system?

My spiritual leader, Dennis Adams, told me one way. It's:

Visually herd all the fears and anxieties you're feeling in this moment into a corral and close the gate.   With them now contained exactly where you visualize them, circle the corral with love, bless all the feelings and release them to God. Sounds funny or too simplistic, but it literally releases them from your system and gives you peace. Yes, it can come back and if it does just do it all over again.

There's another method to release feelings.

How?

I write.

So go grab some paper and a #2 lead pencil. Begin writing. Address your letter to whatever or whoever is involved. As you're writing, don't stop yourself from crying or swearing. Just get it all out. You are alone aren't you? That's exactly what you need. Take the entire page to write one word of anger if you need to. Just let it rip. Do not reread all the hurt and anger you exposed or uncovered by your writing. When you've written (said all you need to say) just burn the paper and let it go. I admit this isn't fun or easy but it does succeed in releasing what you've hidden. If it comes back just do it again. Eventually you will get through. Day by day, little by little it does get easier.

Writing this chapter has ultimately turned out for my greater good. I maintain it was Divine Order. I've accepted this and do acknowledge that Divine Order is showing up in my every day affairs as well even in the little things. Just today my reading glasses caught my attention. I noticed that my fingernail could fit in a small screw in the right arm of my glasses and I could easily turn it. Immediately I went for my jewelry screw driver and tightened it just in time. Thanking my glasses for alerting me I heard, "You're welcome." Imagination?

I'm sure you recognize that we've all looked for love in all the wrong places. As I said before, love can only be found within. Experience has shown and dictated that you cannot give love until you have found and know what love is within yourself.

As soon as you have accepted and felt unconditional love for yourself, then it's very easy to extend unconditional love to others—no attachments—no expected returns—absolutely no hooks—it's FREE.

So be it.

Agreeing brings peace and contentment.

SEVENTEEN

Inner-Feelings:

This subject is way too deep for me. There are too many feelings coming up from Chapter 16. I don't want to address this issue but I must for all of us.

Note: This has actually become more like a personal journal. I make no excuses but don't be surprised at what you are about to read now in Chapter 17. Okay. Let's return and talk about Inner-Feelings.

I have memories of feelings both wonderful and hurtful. My wonderful memories are cherished and I smile and laugh a lot and find I'm delighted to share them. The hurtful ones on the other hand are hidden far, far away. I don't like it at all when they come up and I personally keep those feelings buried deep by eating enough sugar (cookies—candy—cake—pie—donuts—ice cream—etc.) to keep them way down out-of-sight. I never consciously look for them. I know you must understand that.

What would happen if I chose to look at them from a different perspective? What would happen if I brought them forth to the light? What if they were exposed and I allowed myself to feel them? What if I gave up all my sugar addictions and faced myself? Am I willing to admit I am powerless over needing sugar to cover my feelings?

NO WAY! NO WAY AM I DOING THIS! NOT AT ALL!

Having admitted to that, I've been looking at what other things I do besides the immediate huge sugar intake to smooth my inner-feelings away. Here's a big one. I keep all my framed family pictures on my bedroom walls—nothing in the living room, hallways or kitchen. If I receive pictures as snap shots, then they are placed in albums which I never look at. I love it when my kids send me photos by E-mail and I allow myself to gaze at them for a long time smiling all the while before I organize and save them to Drive. But to date I have never reviewed them. Why? Because it hurts me to see pictures of family and they're not here in person. Where are they? Why are visits so few? It's just too sad and lonely. Memories!

Enough about that. I don't like feeling sad and lonely. I want my days to be up-beat. I'm going to stop now and go eat a lot of candy and watch TV. I am. I did.

Observation: (1) My hands are numb (have been for three months now) because I don't want to feel my feelings. The numbness and itching rescinded somewhat in my hands as soon as I was willing to go further. (2) I can only look further into what's happening when I have made myself numb from those same feelings. (3) Not now, but just as soon as this TV program is finished, I'm contacting the Christ within me and asking for what I need to know to be revealed to me.

Yes, I am reluctant and somewhat fearful to proceed.

I'm not really ready. BUT . . . .

I want to eat more sugar right now. Will I? NO, I'll drink some water instead. I will bless the water and ask the water to help me also. I will begin this following mantra saying it out loud continuously over and over again to help calm me before I face myself by writing in my personal journal.

"I love You, God, I love You, God, I love You, God, I love You, God, I love You, God, I love You, God, I love You, God, I love You, God, I love You, God, I love You, God I love You, God, I love You, God, I love You, God, I love You, God, I love You, God."

Note: Instruction on how-to do the mantra: While breathing in say the mantra three times and while expelling your breath out say the mantra three times—breathing in repeating three times and expelling out repeating three times. "I love You, God" three times breathing in and "I love You, God" three times expelling out. Keep this up as long as desired. I didn't time it then but later did and while watching the clock discovered that each "I love You, God" took one second either going in or coming out.

I did the mantra and then went to write in my journal. I received some answers that I believe and trust that they are personal to me and not to be recorded here. So taking in love one more time, I let go of the fear. I stopped, went to rest and let it all soak in.

It's now later in the day @ 7:20 p.m. I've had a substantial dinner--water, meat, potatoes and red cabbage, no dessert. I've been reading a soft cover book—a family fiction about growing grapes and making wine. I'm feeling very emotional. I'm going to do some organizing of my book on ageing and then I'm going to bed. It's 8:00 p.m. I'm still hyper. Recognizing that I still need more relaxing time before sleep, I'm back to reading my fiction story.

Question: Will I ever put this little book up for publication? I have no answer to this question yet. I do know my hands are much better. Are my hands all-tied-together with my feelings? Who knows? I do know I need to connect with my inner voice--the Healing Power within me. I'm ready. I will now proceed to quietly meditate.

IT'S LOVE! I'M HIDING FROM LOVE! Not abandonment. Not rejection. I'm hiding from LOVE.   WHAT LOVE?

I have no words to describe this love that I have needed so desperately. As I search a way to describe what I'm been asking for (the type I never found) there's really only one type of love that I don't already own. That love has to be what I left behind when I chose to be born again into this lifetime. I chose to separate myself from the unconditional love of God—Divine Love. That hurt, that loss of Divine Love was too much to feel so I buried it way down inside.

Realistically I've been told that I've always had it. It's always belonged to me, never left me. I've been aware of that fact for some time already but even then haven't accepted or allowed myself to know it.

An explanation of Divine Love is unconditional love. No judgments—no requirements—no restraints--just completely unconditional. I know I've said this before but it does warrant saying again.

Why did I agree to come back? I think my purpose demands that I be here to help humankind turn away from separation and return to union with God.

ONE. We are only ONE. GOD IS. I AM. YOU ARE.

The joining of love here on earth between two humans is as close to the love of God as we can get. I never found that but did manage to make my peace with it. What I've discovered today is the awareness of the love I left when I chose to return to this earth planet and I repeat:

It's Divine Love I'm asking for.

It's Divine Love I lost when I was re-born here.

It's Divine Love I've always been searching for.

It's Divine Love I open myself to feel now.

Being open and vulnerable is me writing all this. Is that a good thing? I trust it is because it felt right at the moment. It still feels right.

This is a quote from Daily Word, a publication from Unity: "The truth of my being is revealed through spiritual understanding."

Today I encountered an even deeper understanding with God.

"Thank You, God. I am grateful."

EIGHTEEN

Helen's Tuesdays:

Even before first-of-all-tasks, comes talking with God. He's listening I know. And He is reminding me to "Lighten up, Helen". You see, I'm always so serious as if life on this planet is to be taken seriously which isn't exactly true. Life here is meant to learn the truth about myself through relationships and union which means openness and willingness and thinking with my heart.

How I choose to conduct this life is up to me. I want to let it shine the truth of my being. I want to be able to listen to you and see the Christ in you, perfect in every way, so that both you and I can exchange the wonders of this universe and learn about ourselves in a holy encounter. And, oh yes, laugh at ourselves while we learn because we can still be outrageous even though we are Elders in every way.

I'm listening also as I say this: In all things be truthful to yourself as well as to others. Be aware. Allow yourself to be tactful but don't lie. Don't enable.

Does this sound unreal? Am I making it up? Do I have my head in the clouds? Or do I simply want a new life of joy and miracles and peace.

There is an "INVOCATION" in the Book of Runes by Ralph H. Blum which I quote:

> *God within me, God without, How shall I ever be in doubt? There is no place where I may go, And not there see God's face, not know, I am God's vision and God's ear. So through the harvest of my years, I am the Sower and the Sown, God's Self unfolding and God's own."*

Isn't that beautiful? And I look outside off my balcony and see that it is raining, the grass is new and greening and the trees are budding and the birds are singing and life is indeed beautiful.

 Last night in my dreams....

A young mother came to me and was frantic for a place to memorialize her baby's name as he made his transition.   Her frustration became mine. She couldn't find what she so desperately wanted and I was unable to help her so I woke up. Is it not enough that we remember our loved ones in our hearts? Are we not all one? I have no answer. Do you?

Today is a new beginning. A chance to believe in divine guidance in our lives. That we are guided in all we do to our highest good. That we make every decision from our heart staying in this now moment only and not leaning on past experiences or fearful of the future. To know peace, I call upon peace in me first. To know love, I call upon love in me first. To remember my loved ones with joy, I call upon those memories that made me smile. And then I rest knowing that one day we will be together again even as now we are joined in that memory.

If you've noticed I can get on a soapbox very easily. Probably because I was never listened to as a child. We were told that children were to be seen not heard. I really get my head out-of-joint when people interrupt me or second-guess me or top my story. Please excuse me if all of this seems long-winded. BUT I'm passionate about what I'm writing. And no one can interrupt me here. "Thank You, God."

What came up today was a critique that things were not in logical order. I've re-read all this many times and still don't see it. I get carried away and then need to relax a little by turning to something less intense. That's who I am. That's why I skip around. Just bear with me. When I'm factual, that's easy. When I'm emotional or passionate about what I'm writing, that's intense. So be it. This is me being open and truthful.

Words to live by: Appreciation. Gratitude. Thankfulness. Love.

Words from Bill Diedrich. "I am the one who prays. I am the one to whom I pray. I am the one who answers my prayer. God has already answered. It is done. Five Steps: (1) I recognize Divine Mind. (2) I am one with it. (3) I accept healing. (4) Thank You. (5) I let go.

NINETEEN

Exploring Mary's Wisdom:

Life is on-going. We're not meant to give up or stagnate. Hence, I've been out visiting some of my elder friends with questions. They are: "If someone came to you very despondent and frustrated and asked you how to get out of this, what would you answer?" Or…. "If they were very depressed and unable to rise above it, what would you say to them?" Or…. "What are your profound thoughts about age and life? What can you tell me about you? What has had meaning to you?" Here are some answers that they shared with me. With her permission the following comes from my elder friend Mary Menhart,

> "Life doesn't work until you get on a spiritual path. Healing is not about blaming other people for our unhappiness. We have no control over them only ourselves. Every day I ask Holy Spirit to support me in being non-judgmental of others."

> Mary went on, "I didn't want a life of mediocrity. I had strength and faith enough to go and live in Germany without

knowing the language. I learned their language simply by being there and observing their heritage and culture and began to realize that the German people were different in some ways but in all ways still real, kind, meaningful and beautiful. People are people wherever you go and I have traveled and lived in other countries extensively enough to know the truth about that statement. We are all the same underneath regardless of religion or culture or food or life style. And, we all want the same; peace, a decent standard of living, a good education for our children and freedom."

I'm interested in world affairs. I follow the news on TV and keep in touch with the political scene. I like knowing what's going on. "We have to follow our dreams realizing that we are not in control when we see them go in other directions. It's all about trust. Without doubting, we must go with the flow trusting God to know when to proceed, when our perfect time is right. Looking back we might have thought it wrong, we might even have felt angry, until one day we realized that the outcome was better than anticipated or hoped for.

I remember a quote from Robert Browning: "A man's reach should exceed his grasp or what's a heaven for!"

"Thank-you Mary."

Before I left her, she told me she was inspired to begin to write her autobiography that she had always wanted to do so her grandkids would know her. Maybe she would procure a typewriter because it wasn't easy to write long-hand anymore. See, we elders still have spunk and knowledge to share and she honored me by sharing a deeper part of herself which I had never known.

Contemplate this: Every response you make is determined by what you think you are, and what you think you are, and what you want to be, is what you think you are. You may believe that you judge your brothers by the message they give you, but you have judged them by the message you give them.

If a neighbor slights you, don't take it personal. They are hurting in some way. Take a deep breath and look at the situation in another way. Did you approach already on guard or defensive expecting a put-down? Remember that it's never outside yourself.

I firmly believe that God wants us to really, truly, live our lives without fear or regrets. All we have to do is remember that every situation we encounter, even if we view it as bad, is always working out for the common good of all.

TWENTY

Learning Connie's Wisdom:

The following wisdom comes from my elder friend Connie Kupris-Myers. I'm going to mix in a little background here and there as she talks. Just bear with me. Connie is a mother of nine, 3 girls and 6 boys, ranging in current age from 68 to 48. She told me her advice to them was "Be kind to others and make me proud." Widowed twice she raised her children Catholic. She herself is now a Unity of Grand Rapids student and member. Connie just lost her youngest daughter, Brenda, at the age of 48 to cancer.

> She says today (two months later), "I feel guilty putting her death out of my mind. But I want to remember her with joy and not continue feeling sad. That's because my basic belief is that laughter brings and maintains a happy, calm life. When each of my husbands died, I knew I had to start making a new life because I still had my children to raise and regardless of circumstances, I must go on. Losing my daughter is different. She was brave and

never admitted to pain or let any of us know she was disheartened—not to me and certainly not to her own kids. She didn't share, complain or talk about it. She only acknowledged a positive outcome and she always had music playing. And of course, we all supported her wish to remain peaceful and happy and hopeful. It only lasted a short six months from the first prognosis. She didn't give up until her cousin came to say goodbye. Within a week after that she was admitted to hospice on a Sunday evening and made a peaceful transition the very next Thursday morning.

I have really learned a few things about grief that I feel are important. One is a friend called me within two days after Brenda died and I cried all the time she was on the phone with me. It meant so much that she called me right away and was able and willing to acknowledge and share what I was going through. So, DO NOT HESITATE TO REACH OUT IMMEDIATELY. I felt blessed and really appreciated it.

Here's something else that has just come along. I was reading Facebook and saw this little quote that someone had written about grief. It really captured my attention. I thought, "Oh my God," this is what grief is all about. I copied it and want to share it with my family. It helped me so much. I hope it helps them too.

Grief never ends but it changes.
It's a passage, not a place to stay.
Grief is not a sign of weakness,
Nor a lack of faith.
It is the price of Love."

How do I survive day to day? It's like a bad dream so I put it out of my mind because dreams can be forgotten. Right? I think that's how I've reacted my entire adult life. My life must be happy and content because I simply can't function in sadness. If sadness was what was going on, I would think of things I did before that I could laugh about. And that's true even today. I like to lighten up the mood. You may think I'm devilish but I'm not. I simply say outrageous things to change the feeling around me. Something risqué like, "I don't ever gaze at a man's butt. I look at his zipper!" Are you laughing? So am I and it always does change the atmosphere. I like to say things that are shocking to get attention. (Is that my ego talking?) I'm really pretty straight-laced. I just like to joke. Believe it or not, I was quiet and serious as a kid but not anymore.

I like things simple but organized so that I can say, "Whatever will be will be." It's not my way to say that it's Divine Order. That's too churchy. But I am willing to acknowledge contentment and peace when I'm being in *agreement* with where I'm at. (Don't give me away but those are Helen's words.)

Every morning now I get up and see the bright side as much as I can because I want to remember Brenda with joy not sorrow. I want to be loving and to have a happy frame of mind and be at peace with my life. If I was to write my own epitaph it would be my motto, IT IS WHAT IT IS. "

"Thank you, Connie."

TWENTY ONE

Discovering Bethy's Wisdom:

Let me Introduce you to my elder friend Bethy Shaw. This is a woman who remembers every one of us every day in her morning prayers. She visualizes us and repeats our name as she touches each bead on her rosary. If you look like you need a prayer, you've got it. If it's a situation that needs prayer, it's done. No matter how big or how small, here is someone on this planet who remembers to go to God. She asks always for our highest good and her prayers all end with "Not my will but thine be done."

> Bethy says, "I'm here to be human. God is me—living in me. My ego is who I am, being my humanity. Being who I am, I recognize the love in me and that it needs passing on. I live my life to please others and that feels good to me and makes me complete. Family is important. It's okay to cry if I'm missing them because sometimes I just need to let them go.
>
> I'm very sedentary, always have been. I've never felt real healthy and hate bending

over. That's why I don't garden. Joy things to me are reading, watching TV, using my computer, phoning friends and playing my piano.

I do love writing letters or sending little notes that let other friends, friends who also can't get around, know that I care. Sometimes the letters or notes only say something personal or let's pretend like; I've just invited you to join me on my porch to have a spot of tea and watch the birds. One of my friends actually answered me just to say how much she loved the letters because she could save them and read them over and over again making them a continued pleasure.

In my 50's and 60's I belonged to a group (bi-racial—both sexes) dedicated to make people happy called Curtain-Time-Players. We composed and acted in skits, built our own props and costumes, switched roles as needed and performed to various groups all over town. What fun it was.

I like to make people happy. My days are filled thinking of what I can do tomorrow to make someone happy. I share jokes all the time so we can laugh together. Risqué jokes are the best. I admit that I want everyone to love me. I shy away from anger because I don't have the courage to confront.

I don't trust easily. I'm still working on that. I value my independence and am deeply grateful that I can still manage my own affairs and my life. I believe that all religions lead us to God and that every person has the right to choose the perfect path that is meant for them to follow. I'm not afraid to die but I am afraid of the dying process. My goal and my motto has always been to make people happy and to simply be the God that I am.

"Thank you, Bethy."

Two of these elder friends mention they are not afraid to die but are afraid of the dying process. I think that's true of most of us but how I think I'll act and how I will act maybe entirely different. The best way I know how to overcome fear is to trust all the times we've been told to let the fear go. Putting ourselves in *agreement* and believing in Divine Order helps to lesson that fear. Our true self had always been connected to God. Only our thoughts have kept us separated from Him and in death we will simply be returning home.

Like the story of the prodigal son, our Father awaits us with joy and eagerly welcomes us with open arms.

You'll note that I've only interviewed elders. Please don't take offense. We are all the same ONE. There is no time proclaiming one age wiser than another. It's simply because this is where I am. My ego (Yes, I admit it) says, "Look at me. I want you to recognize I'm still alive and kicking. And you, my readers say back to me, "But the wise don't need to think it or proclaim it. It just is. Look at the words of wisdom that are coming out of our little ones. They simply know."

I've noticed these attributes in elders that I see. If they have courage, they are empowered. If they are fearless, they are strong. If they are listeners, they are fulfilled. If they are quiet, there is inner wisdom. If they are open, they see life with eyes of joy.

TWENTY TWO

An Elder's Take:

The ups and downs of being an Elder are typical. Each side is equal in intensity. For instance: Strength—Weakness; Hot—Cold; Childlike— Sage wisdom;   Help me—Don't touch me; Please come in—Go away; Yes, I will—No, I won't.

I'm exhausted from what this balancing act requires. Never-the-less my Energy/Activity Chart still has to be recognized and todays EAC is very different.

For instance, now 4 months short of 91 years old:

I've used most of my energy lately composing and finalizing this book	3-8 points
I've cut back on card game and keeping score	0-2 points
Jig-saw puzzles: 300 piece/easy, 500/ok, 750/hard, 1000/forget it	1-3 points

2 Unity classes on Thursdays (drive-class-lunch-class-drive)	6-7 points
Driving my car every 20 miles	1 point
I find my best energy in the mornings. That's when I do the necessary heavy activities: grocery shopping	2-3 points
or laundry/changing bedding	3-5 points

I have help cleaning. All other activities need to be fitted in like doctor visits. So I relax with lunches out, watching TV and reading paperback fiction stories.

Exercise and walking takes me longer now as I go slower and don't do as much. I consider this filling in the day by taking-a-break or changing-my-mood.

Activities previously listed seem to be free and easy—almost zero energy needed. Full days like the Unity classes require resting days both before and after.

My days really vary and I can't actually make a chart. Never-the-less I recognize that I still need to hold myself to a range of activity between 7-8-9 and still need to watch my energy intake especially making sure I eat something timely and drink plenty of water. I get excited about writing. Going overboard seems to be the norm because I'm on a roll and I don't want to stop. Whenever this happens I simply take a half-hour nap. (No pain anymore at all. Isn't that great?)

Creative thoughts come at odd moments and must be written down immediately or they are lost. Sometimes I'm up two or three hours during the night because I'm either composing (writing it down) or typing on my laptop. Some days this little book is all I do. I try to keep Tuesdays and Fridays free for just that. Does it work? Not quite always but pretty much. My days are over-flowing. Sometimes I'm thrilled. Sometimes I'm tickled. Sometimes I'm frustrated. Sometimes I'm very pleased but always I'm able to say "Thank You, God".

> *Agreeing* with my life as it is now, I affirm wholeness and strength. I am rejuvenated and restored.

> *Agreeing* has me acknowledging my value.

Agreeing encourages dream accomplishment.

This book started out with tricks to *agreeing with ageing.* If you've noticed previous intense core issues of mine have turned up from the easiest to the deepest and materialized in chapters. In between I hope you found a few informative chapters placed strategically.

The world we live in is a learning process. We look, we watch, we absorb, we apply what we see to our present circumstances. We have been taught to look outside ourselves for answers. If this way doesn't work then show me, better yet, teach me a new way and I will put it into effect. This is a pattern of looking without and wondering what to do about what we see rather than a pattern of looking within and changing what we see. It literally points out we do not trust ourselves but think the next person knows more than we do.

The truth is that we do know, we just don't know that we know.

STOP IT.   WE ARE POWERFUL.   ALL OF US.

EPILOGUE

Agreeing is still the price of ageing.

Agreeing with age is like applying a clothes softener sheet to your life. It softens the wrinkles—reduces static cling and freshens the air.

Agreeing with age lightens its many loads, let's your mind lift to light.

Agreeing with age brings this day into focus without any blinders of regret.

Agreeing with age brings a happy ending to whatever fear is facing you.

We have no other choice but to *agree* if we want to live in peace. We cannot live in conflict every moment—disagreeing with every opportunity— fearful to change—hiding. That *agreeing* word can be interpreted in other ways as evidenced by what you beheld as you read how these three other elders live their lives.

Is contentment your only goal? Do you want more? Then reach out. Try something new. Dare yourself and wake up that imagination of yours. LIVE! Whatever is your secret, uncover it. Share it. God means us to mingle, to listen, to learn and to love one another.

If I remember correctly, the Mama Eagle bird gradually removes the comfort elements from the nest leaving only prickly, sharp thorns to encourage her babies to give up, let go, try their wings and FLY. This is a lesson for us too. So be it.

What we think—what we say—becomes real. "And the word was made flesh." Remember that Bible message? Look within. Accept the new. Meet each day with courage, determination and confidence.

Hebrew scriptures share this reminder "Keep your heart with all vigilance, for from it flows the springs of life." This came from Daily Word.

"There are two ways to live your life. One is as though nothing is a miracle. The other is as though everything is a miracle." -— Albert Einstein. A quote from (CIM) Miracles magazine.

Resisting is the opposite of *agreeing*. When we cease to struggle against our age is when we begin to enjoy our age. As a swimmer I learned to float in the water as soon as I stopped resisting and relaxed enough to let the water hold me. It was that accomplishment that eventually turned into swimming. What a happy day.

Isn't that the same way we began to know God?

STAY POSITIVE. Remind yourself of your past successes and picture yourself being active again. Don't expect perfection. If today you get off track know you can always get back on. Finding balance in life is a skill. Harmony and balance are one. So within—so without. If you think you can, you can. Even at our age we are still worthy and needed.

Just put yourself in *agreement*.   Live in the NOW. Believe in Divine Order. Give yourself credit when you recognize a new phase and are able to let it go.

Be aware that you and I have the ability and the power to change our thoughts, perspectives and habits. And that changing an attitude involves a renewed commitment to self-care, to provide our bodies with adequate rest, nourishment and encouragement. Don't forget an apple a day keeps the doctor away.

Find yourself. Together we can do this. Stay well! Stay happy!   Try *Agreeing*!   Enjoy!

Blessings on you and all that you see!

Thanks for reading,

Helen

References:

Dennis Adams, Spiritual Leader and Healer:

> contactus@dennisadamsmasterhealer.com

Daily Word, a Unity Publication:

> dailyword.com   -and-
> unity.org/communities

Bill Diedrich, Speaker, Writer, Teacher:

> theroadhome@comcast.net

A Course In Miracles (CIM):

> www.miraclesmagazine.org

A Course Of Love:

> www.acourseoflove.org

www.ingramcontent.com/pod-product-compliance
Lightning Source LLC
Chambersburg PA
CBHW020326290526
45785CB00007B/2938